Air Fryer Cookbook for Beginners

Easy, Healthy & Low Carb Recipes That Will Help Keep You Sane

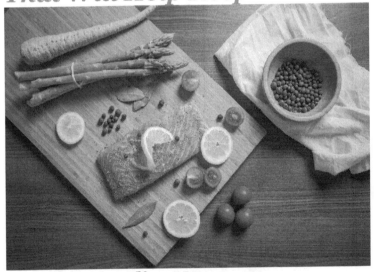

Alice Newman

ISBN-13:978-1724442963

ISBN-10:1724442961

Table of Contents

ISBN-13:978-1724442963

ISBN-10:1724442961

Introduction

Thank you so much for purchasing *Air Fryer Cookbook for Beginners*!

This is no ordinary cookbook, however. While this book is loaded with recipes that are low carb, low in bad fats and full of healthy high fat ingredients, also that are low-sodium, there is a special twist that makes this cookbook even healthier than those other diet fads out there among the masses. I am pleased to introduce you to the air fryer! This kitchen gadget can cook your everyday favorites with just the circulation of hot air. If you are someone that is always disappointed by a lack of crispiness in their food, then the air fryer is the appliance for you!

You have purchased a cookbook that not only has a wide variety of delectable and easy-to-make air fryer recipes but one that holds an entire chapter dedicated to helping you fuel your body in a healthier manner, as well as a chapter loaded with tips to get the most out of your air fryer experience! I would also say that these recipes would help to keep your keto diet every day.

While there are hundreds of cookbooks on the market today, I want to thank you again for choosing this air fryer cookbook. You have made a great choice and will not be disappointed! Every effort was made to ensure it is full of as much useful information as possible, please enjoy!

Eating Healthy in a World of Temptation

We all know it, and you are here because you know it too; eating healthy is not only a fad choice but an entire change to your lifestyle and state of mind.

Each day you must strive to make good decisions and take baby steps towards your fitness goals. Slowly but surely, you seem to create healthy habits that stick.

But in the world, we live in today, there is literally temptation around every corner. From the candy bowl at work to the restaurant menu to the fast food joint perfectly stationed on your commute home, it is hard to say no to such delicious enticements. So, how is one supposed to fortify themselves to stay on track?

This chapter will discuss some of the best tips to assist you in achieving your fitness goals, whether you wish to shed some excess fat or are just wanting to look and feel a bit better, there is always a way to shield yourself against unhealthy temptations.

Eat before you go

It is difficult to make healthy decisions when your stomach is growling.

Make sure you eat before you head to work, to the store, or anywhere where you might be led to make a poor choice in food.

Or, take a healthy snack with you. If you are always letting yourself get to the point of "hangry-ness," you are blatantly setting yourself up to feast in the land of junk foods.

It is also important to eat consistent meals throughout the day to help you stay on track as well. Learn to cook in the comfort of your own home instead of wasting your hard-earned money on food that really doesn't suit you well.

Plan ahead

It is in your best interest to be prepared. Start each week by making yourself a meal plan. List what you need and make it a goal to stick as close as you can to this plan. This will help you to reduce the number of times you go to the store, which results in a decrease of impulsive buys.

Plan for dining out too! Many restaurants now post their entire menu online for customers to look at. Know what options they have available, which will make it easier to make healthier decisions.

Trick what triggers you

All of us have a version of kryptonite, those delicious but bad-for-you eats that leave us feeling helpless and unable to fight back.

Keep these sorts of temptations out of sight and out of mind, or better yet, out of your home and office altogether.

To stay the course of becoming a healthier version of yourself, you must learn the importance of making decisions when confronted with healthier alternatives to what you are triggered by to counteract them.

For example, if you are like me, ice cream is always a losing battle. Instead of heading to scoop some mint chocolate chip that is loaded with sugar and countless calories, opt to make a healthier version, such as Banana Ice Cream!

Investigate cravings

When you find yourself in a hankering for something unsavory for your body, take a moment to stop and ask yourself *why* you are craving a certain item. What is it that you are craving? There are many of us, myself included, that mix up our emotional cravings with food, and sadly, food will never fill this type of void.

If you are always falling for some sort of temptation, look inside yourself and consider what your energy is like and what you are feeling and thinking at that moment. People are more prone to unhealthy and overeating when they are stressed out, tired, anxious, bored, or trying to cope with an uncertain situation. Instead of using food to cope, evaluate your emotional status and see how you can resolve the negativity that is fueling your bad choice making when it comes to what you eat and what you crave.

Create a path to success

Make it a priority to keep up with a food journal. Track what you eat, how you feel when you eat items, what makes you crave certain things, etc. Often, simply jotting down a terrible choice of food can lead you to make much better decisions in the future.

You can also write out mantras in this journal as well. Make up a phrase you can easily remember that will help you to find the motivation to keep moving forward in a healthy pattern.

- "I'm worth it."
- "I am striving for ultimate health."
- "I am in control of the choices I make."

Act on "give-ins" in moderation

It is perfectly fine to give in and succumb to our favorite junk foods that ultimately satisfy our taste buds on occasion. Make sure to write down your cravings in your food journal. I like to tell people to eat for fuel 90% of the time and eat for fun 10%!

Don't stop

Don't let an occasional slip-up detour you from sticking to your goal of becoming a healthier version of yourself. We are all human and make mistakes.

Don't get all caught up in eating something unhealthy and ruin your day because of it. You have the control to turn that once unhealthy day into a very healthy one.

Let carbs fight for you

Anti-carb attitudes are wildly outdated. Research has shown how carbohydrates that are packed with resistant starches can help you to feel more satisfied and promote overall satiety. It takes energy to break down these starches and causes a decrease in insulin spikes compared to "bad carbs."

Believe it or not, carbs are essential to the weight loss game. If you eat more healthy carbs and avoid the processed ones, you are giving your body the energy source it needs and prefers, which provides you with the ultimate mental satisfaction you need to keep pushing forward.

Get grateful

When you are famished, and at home alone, it can be very tempting to grab that bag of mini donuts to nom on instead of picking a piece of fruit. Before you decide on s snack, take a moment to pause and appreciate.

Ponder over how hard it is to grow produce to eat, how much you enjoy the natural juiciness of biting into an orange, or walking to the farmers market. Can you say any of these things about that bag of mini donuts you were about to devour?

Gratitude is one of those off-key things that can ultimately help you in your weight loss and fitness journey. You are taking a second to find the foods that bring your nourishment, which is a lot harder to come by with processed eats. This helps in the decision process of making thoughtful choices.

Don't fear these foods

Despite what many people think and what you have read time after time, the following foods at great if you are striving for a finer waistline!

- *Cereal and milk*: While there are many cereals out there that are packed with excess sugars with barely any nutritional value, there are many others that have 2 ½ grams of fiber per serving. Eat these types with 8 ounces of whole milk to feel satisfied in the morning. Opt for cereals that have 10 grams or less of sugar per serving. If you are hankering for additional sweetness, eat a piece of fruit!

- *Greek yogurt*: Opt for whole-milk Greek yogurt, and you will get a healthy source of fat that satiates you! Eating high-fat dairy items can help in lowering the risk of becoming overweight by 8%.

- *Dried fruits*: While many people think that dried fruit is as bad for you as gummy candies are, this is simply not true. While you should never overeat dried fruit, these are not packed with added sugars and is denser in calories than raw fruit. Loaded with vitamins and fiber, it can make a great snack in moderation.

- *White potatoes:* Known for their high carbohydrate content, many people try their best to avoid white potatoes. But it isn't their carb content as much as it is the forms we eat them in. From potato chips to fries drizzled with butter, it is no wonder these below ground veggies have gotten a bad rap. Potatoes, when not covered in processed things, are packed with potassium, full of vitamins and are relatively low in calorie count. They are good carbs and increase overall satiety.

Don't force foods you hate on yourself

Do not feel bad if you are not with your friends and coworkers on hopping on the newest and latest diet fads. This certainly does not mean you are on the wrong track. If there are certain foods you do not like and appreciate, then don't force yourself to eat them.

This will only detour you from sticking to your health goals. It will leave you more unsatisfied than before, and you will feel less nourished.

How to Plan Your Low Carb Diet

To achieve weight loss, you will need to reduce your carbohydrate intake. You will soon realize the plan will allow you to feel full and satisfied while still dropping the pounds. You restrict carb intake in your diet which includes starches such as bread and pasta as well as sugars. Because of the keto diet, you will replace them with fat and protein. Not only will you lose weight; you will also lower blood pressure, triglycerides, and blood sugar.

What works for one person as a 'low-carb' diet may be too low for another person. It depends on your activity levels, age, body composition, and gender. It may also depend on your metabolic health, food culture, and personal preferences. If you are more active and have more muscle mass; you can tolerate more carbs versus someone who is sedentary. If people get the metabolic syndrome, he/she may become obese or suffer from type II diabetes whereas the rules change. It is sometimes referred to by the scientists as 'carbohydrate intolerance.'

As mentioned, there's no set rule for carb intake. These are some of the basic guidelines to consider as you blaze the path on the ketogenic diet plan which is effective about 90% of the time. By using the Instant Pot with the plan, you will soon see results in much less time. Use the carbs wisely.

Beginning with the most difficult phase of the ketogenic plan:

20-50 Grams Daily

Losing weight falls into this category. If you have are obese, diabetes, or metabolically deranged, this is the plan for you. If you are consuming less than the 50 grams daily; your body will achieve a ketosis state which supplies the ketone bodies.

Consider these guidelines:

- Some berries with whipped cream
- Plenty of low-carbohydrate veggies
- Trace carbs from foods including nuts, seeds, and avocados

50-100 Grams Daily:

- Plenty of veggies
- 2-3 pieces of fruit each day
- Minimal intake of starchy carbs

Moderate Carb Intake: 100-150 Grams Daily

If you are active and lean trying to maintain weight, these are some of the foods to consider:

- Several fruits daily
- All the veggies you can eat
- Healthy starches such as rice, oats, sweet potatoes, and potatoes

As you now see, it is important to experiment and categorize where you fall on the scales before you make any changes. Seek your doctor's advice before changing your eating patterns. In some cases, you could reduce the need for some medications.

Getting the Most Out of Your Air Fryer

If those tips in the last chapter weren't awesome enough on their own, I am pleased to introduce you to an appliance that can help you to trick those cravings! If you are a fan of fried foods, (I mean, who *isn't*?!) then this nifty kitchen appliance will help you to feel more satisfied by what you eat by helping you to whip up healthier versions of your favorite cheat snacks and meals!

What is an Air Fryer?

Air fryers work by cooking food with the circulation of hot air. This is what makes the foods you put into it so crispy when they come out! Something called the "Maillard Effect" happens, which is a chemically induced reaction that occurs to the heat that makes it capable for this fryer to brown foods in such a short time, while keeping nutrients *and* flavor intact.

To dumb it down, air fryers can do what those oil fryers do, but in a much healthier way than submerging food into greasy and fattening oil.

Benefits of Using an Air Fryer

Since the air fryer takes away the need to use all that excess oil, there are a plethora of health benefits you can receive by using it to cook everyday meals and snacks:

- Less calories that can lead to weight gain and obesity
- Decreased risk of high blood pressure
- Decreased risk of heart disease and clogged arteries
- Decreased risk of having a stroke or an aneurysm

Pros and Cons of the Air Fryer

Pros:

- Much faster than regular frying alternatives
- Versatile; can be used to bake, grill, roast, and more!
- Easy to clean, thanks to the use of little oil

Obviously, air fryers are a much healthier alternative to oil frying. However, there are a few cons to consider if you are thinking about getting one of your very own:

Cons:

- Are small and don't have a ton of room to cook items
- Bulky and heavy in nature, even though capacity is rather small
- Can get extremely hot, but not as dangerous as traditional oil fryers.

Tips to Use Air Fryer

Air fryers can give you crispier foods that satisfy your cravings. Here are some great tips for you to get the most out of your air fryer!

Shake it!

Be sure to open the fryer and shake what you are cooking around as they "fry" in the basket. Smaller foods such as French fries and chips may compress. Even if a recipe does not mention to rotate, shake, or flip, for the best results, make sure to do so every 5-10 minutes.

Do not overcrowd

Make sure you give foods lots of space for the hot air to circulate effectively around what you are cooking. This will give you the crispy results you crave! Also, it is best to work in small batches.

Spray foods

Most recipes will tell you to do such, but if not, it is a good idea to lightly spray foods with a bit of oil, so they do not stick to the basket as they cook. I suggest investing in a kitchen spray bottle to put oil in. Much easier to spray foods, so you don't totally saturate them with this greasy stuff.

Keep dry

Make sure you pat foods dry before adding them to air fryer basket. This helps to prevent splattering and excess smoking. So, let marinated foods drip a bit before adding and make sure to empty the fat from the bottom of the fryer when you are done cooking foods that are high in fat content.

Master other methods of cooking

The air fryer is not just for frying! It is great for other methods of cooking, such as grilling, roasting, and even baking! It is my go-to appliance to get the best-tasting salmon!

Add water when cooking fatty foods

Add water to the drawer underneath the basket will help to prevent the grease in fattier foods from becoming too hot and causing smoke to engulf your kitchen. Do this with burgers, sausage, and bacon especially.

Hold foods down with toothpicks

On occasion, your air fryer will pick up foods that are light and blow them around the fryer. Secure foods you cook with toothpicks!

Open as often as you like

One of the best benefits of cooking with an air fryer is that you do not have to worry about how often you open it up to check for doneness.

If you are an anxious chef, this can give you peace of mind to create yummy meals and snacks every single time!

Take out basket before removing food

If you go to invert the air fryer basket when it is still locked tightly in the drawer, you will dump all the fat that has rendered from your food.

Clean the drawer after each use

The air fryer drawer is extremely easy to clean and quite hassle-free. But if you leave it unwashed, you can risk contaminating future food you cook, and you may have a nasty smell takeover your kitchen. Simply clean it after *every* use to prevent this.

Use the air dryer to dry the appliance out

After you wash the basket and air fryer drawer, you can pop them back into the fryer and turn on the appliance for 2-3 minutes. This is a great way to thoroughly dry it for your next use!

Vegetable Recipes

Air Fryer Asparagus

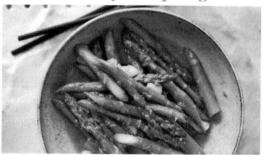

Calories: 17 Fat: 4g Protein: 9g Sugar: 0g Servings: 2

Ingredients:

- Nutritional yeast
- Olive oil non-stick spray
- One bunch of asparagus

Directions:

1. Wash asparagus and then trim off thick, woody ends.

2. Spray asparagus with olive oil spray and sprinkle with yeast.

3. In your air fryer, lay asparagus in a singular layer.

4. Cook 8 minutes at 360 degrees.

Spicy Sweet Potato Fries

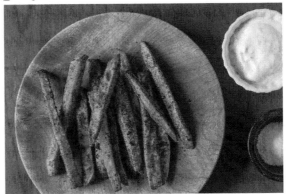

Calories: 89 Fat: 14g   Protein: 8g Sugar: 3g
Prep: 20 minutes
Servings: 4

Ingredients:

- 2 tbsp. sweet potato fry seasoning mix
- 2 tbsp. olive oil
- 2 sweet potatoes

Seasoning Mix:

- 2 tbsp. salt
- 1 tbsp. cayenne pepper
- 1 tbsp. dried oregano
- 1 tbsp. fennel
- 2 tbsp. coriander

Directions:

1. Slice both ends off sweet potatoes and peel. Slice lengthwise in half and again crosswise to make four pieces from each potato.

2. Slice each potato piece into 2-3 slices, then slice into fries.

3. Grind together all of seasoning mix ingredients and mix in the salt.

4. Ensure air fryer is preheated to 350 degrees.

5. Toss potato pieces in olive oil, sprinkling with seasoning mix and tossing well to coat thoroughly.

6. Add fries to air fryer basket and set time for 27 minutes. Press start and cook 15 minutes.

7. Take out the basket and turn fries. Turn off air fryer and let cook 10-12 minutes till fries are golden.

Air Fryer Cauliflower Rice

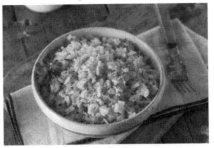

Calories: 67 Fat: 8g Protein: 3g Sugar: 0g
Prep: 20 minutes
Servings: 2-4

Ingredients:

Round 1:

- 1 tsp. turmeric
- 1 C. diced carrot
- ½ C. diced onion
- 2 tbsp. low-sodium soy sauce
- ½ block of extra firm tofu

Round 2:

- ½ C. frozen peas
- 2 minced garlic cloves
- ½ C. chopped broccoli
- 1 tbsp. minced ginger
- 1 tbsp. rice vinegar
- 1 ½ tsp. toasted sesame oil
- 2 tbsp. reduced-sodium soy sauce
- 3 C. riced cauliflower

Directions:

1. Crumble tofu in a large bowl and toss with all the Round one ingredients.
2. Preheat air fryer to 370 degrees and cook 10 minutes, making sure to shake once.
3. In another bowl, toss ingredients from Round 2 together.
4. Add Round 2 mixture to air fryer and cook another 10 minutes, ensuring to shake 5 minutes in.
5. Enjoy!

Air Fried Carrots, Yellow Squash & Zucchini

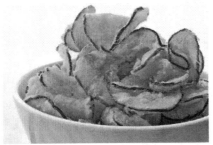

Calories: 122 Fat: 9g Protein: 6g Sugar: 0g
Prep: 7 minutes
Servings: 4

Ingredients:

- 1 tbsp. chopped tarragon leaves
- ½ tsp. white pepper
- 1 tsp. salt
- 1 pound yellow squash
- 1 pound zucchini
- 6 tsp. olive oil
- ½ pound carrots

Directions:

1. Stem and root the end of squash and zucchini and cut in ¾-inch half-moons. Peel and cut carrots into 1-inch cubes

2. Combine carrot cubes with 2 teaspoons of olive oil, tossing to combine. Pour into air fryer basket and cook 5 minutes at 400 degrees.

3. As carrots cook, drizzle remaining olive oil over squash and zucchini pieces, then season with pepper and salt. Toss well to coat.

4. Add squash and zucchini when the timer for carrots goes off. Cook 30 minutes, making sure to toss 2-3 times during the cooking process.

5. Once done, take out veggies and toss with tarragon. Serve up warm!

Air Fried Kale Chips

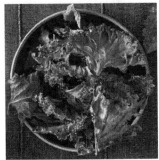

Calories: 55 Fat: 10g Protein: 1g Sugar: 0g
Prep: 5 minutes
Servings: 4-6

Ingredients:

- ¼ tsp. Himalayan salt
- 3 tbsp. yeast
- Avocado oil
- 1 bunch of kale

Directions:

1. Rinse kale and with paper towels, dry well.
2. Tear kale leaves into large pieces. Remember they will shrink as they cook so good sized pieces are necessary.
3. Place kale pieces in a bowl and spritz with avocado oil till shiny. Sprinkle with salt and yeast.
4. With your hands, toss kale leaves well to combine.
5. Pour half of the kale mixture into air fryer. Cook 5 minutes at 350 degrees. Remove and repeat with another half of kale.

Cheesy Cauliflower Fritters

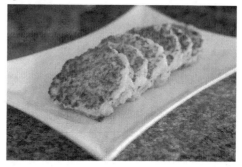

Calories: 209 Fat: 17g Protein: 6g Sugar: 0.5g
Prep: 5 minutes
Servings: 8

Ingredients:

- ½ C. chopped parsley
- 1 C. Italian breadcrumbs
- 1/3 C. shredded mozzarella cheese
- 1/3 C. shredded sharp cheddar cheese
- 1 egg
- 2 minced garlic cloves
- 3 chopped scallions
- 1 head of cauliflower

Directions:

- Cut cauliflower up into florets. Wash well and pat dry. Place into a food processor and pulse 20-30 seconds till it looks like rice.

- Place cauliflower rice in a bowl and mix with pepper, salt, egg, cheeses, breadcrumbs, garlic, and scallions.
- With hands, form 15 patties of the mixture. Add more breadcrumbs if needed.
- With olive oil, spritz patties, and place into your air fryer in a single layer.
- Cook 14 minutes at 390 degrees, flipping after 7 minutes.

Avocado Fries

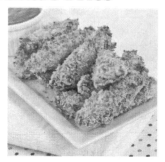

Calories: 102 Fat: 22g Protein: 9g Sugar: 1g
Prep: 5 minutes
Servings: 6

Ingredients:

- 1 avocado
- ½ tsp. salt
- ½ C. panko breadcrumbs
- Bean liquid (aquafaba) from a 15-ounce can of white or garbanzo beans

Directions:

- Peel, pit, and slice up avocado.
- Toss salt and breadcrumbs together in a bowl. Place aquafaba into another bowl.
- Dredge slices of avocado first in aquafaba and then in panko, making sure you get an even coating.
- Place coated avocado slices into a single layer in the air fryer.
- Cook 5 minutes at 390 degrees, shaking at 5 minutes.
- Serve with your favorite keto dipping sauce!

Zucchini Parmesan Chips

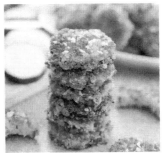

Calories: 211 Fat: 16g Protein: 8g Sugar: 0g
Prep: 5 minutes
Servings: 10

Ingredients:

- ½ tsp. paprika
- ½ C. grated parmesan cheese
- ½ C. Italian breadcrumbs
- 1 lightly beaten egg
- 2 thinly sliced zucchinis

Directions:

- Use a very sharp knife or mandolin slicer to slice zucchini as thinly as you can. Pat off extra moisture.
- Beat egg with a pinch of pepper and salt and a bit of water.
- Combine paprika, cheese, and breadcrumbs in a bowl.

- Dip slices of zucchini into the egg mixture and then into breadcrumb mixture. Press gently to coat.
- With olive oil cooking spray, mist coated zucchini slices. Place into your air fryer in a single layer.
- Cook 8 minutes at 350 degrees.
- Sprinkle with salt and serve with salsa.

Crispy Roasted Broccoli

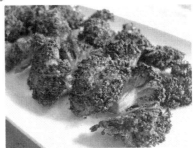

Calories: 96 Fat: 1.3g Protein: 7g Sugar: 4.5g
Prep: 45 minutes
Servings: 2

Ingredients:

- ¼ tsp. Masala
- ½ tsp. red chili powder
- ½ tsp. salt
- ¼ tsp. turmeric powder
- 1 tbsp. chickpea flour
- 2 tbsp. yogurt
- 1 pound broccoli

Directions:

- Cut broccoli up into florets. Soak in a bowl of water with 2 teaspoons of salt for at least half an hour to remove impurities.
- Take out broccoli florets from water and let drain. Wipe down thoroughly.

- Mix all other ingredients together to create a marinade.
- Toss broccoli florets in the marinade. Cover and chill 15-30 minutes.
- Preheat air fryer to 390 degrees. Place marinated broccoli florets into the fryer. Cook 10 minutes.
- 5 minutes into cooking shake the basket. Florets will be crispy when done.

Crispy Jalapeno Coins

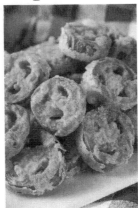

Calories: 128 Fat: 8g Protein: 7g Sugar: 0g
Prep: 10 minutes
Servings: 8-10

Ingredients:

- 1 egg
- 2-3 tbsp. coconut flour
- 1 sliced and seeded jalapeno
- Pinch of garlic powder
- Pinch of onion powder
- Pinch of Cajun seasoning (optional)
- Pinch of pepper and salt

Directions:

- Ensure your air fryer is preheated to 400 degrees.
- Mix together all dry ingredients.
- Pat jalapeno slices dry. Dip coins into egg wash and then into dry mixture. Toss to thoroughly coat.
- Add coated jalapeno slices to air fryer in a singular layer. Spray with olive oil.
- Cook just till crispy.

Buffalo Cauliflower

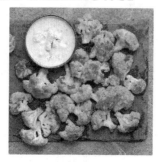

Calories: 194 Fat: 17g Protein: 10g Sugar: 3g
Prep: 15 minutes
Servings: 6-8

Ingredients:

Cauliflower:
- 1 C. panko breadcrumbs
- 1 tsp. salt
- 4 C. cauliflower florets

Buffalo Coating:
- ¼ C. Vegan Buffalo sauce
- ¼ C. melted vegan butter

Directions:
- Melt butter in microwave and whisk in buffalo sauce.
- Dip each cauliflower floret into buffalo mixture, ensuring it gets coated well. Hold over a bowl till floret is done dripping.
- Mix breadcrumbs with salt.

- Dredge dipped florets into breadcrumbs and place into air fryer.
- Cook 14-17 minutes at 350 degrees. When slightly browned, they are ready to eat!
- Serve with your favorite keto dipping sauce!

Jicama Fries

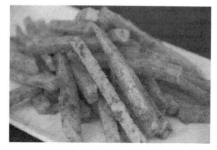

Calories: 211 Fat: 19g Protein: 9g Sugar: 1g
Prep: 10 minutes
Servings: 8

Ingredients:
- 1 tbsp. dried thyme
- ¾ C. arrowroot flour
- ½ large Jicama
- 2 eggs

Directions:
- Sliced jicama into fries.

- Whisk eggs together and pour over fries. Toss to coat.

- Mix a pinch of salt, thyme, and arrowroot flour together. Toss egg-coated jicama into dry mixture, tossing to coat well.

- Spray air fryer basket with olive oil and add fries. Cook 20 minutes on CHIPS setting. Toss halfway into the cooking process.

Air Fryer Brussels Sprouts

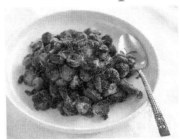

Calories: 118 Fat: 9g Protein: 11g Sugar: 1g
Prep: 5 minutes
Servings: 5

Ingredients:
- ¼ tsp. salt
- 1 tbsp. balsamic vinegar
- 1 tbsp. olive oil
- 2 C. Brussels sprouts

Directions:
- Cut Brussels sprouts in half lengthwise. Toss with salt, vinegar, and olive oil till coated thoroughly.

- Add coated sprouts to air fryer, cooking 8-10 minutes at 400 degrees. Shake after 5 minutes of cooking.

- Brussels sprouts are ready to devour when brown and crisp!

Spaghetti Squash Tots

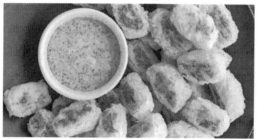

Calories: 231 Fat: 18g Protein: 5g Sugar: 0g
Prep: 5 minutes
Servings: 8-10

Ingredients:

- ¼ tsp. pepper
- ½ tsp. salt
- 1 thinly sliced scallion
- 1 spaghetti squash

Directions:

- Wash and cut the squash in half lengthwise. Scrape out the seeds.
- With a fork, remove spaghetti meat by strands and throw out skins.
- In a clean towel, toss in squash and wring out as much moisture as possible. Place in a bowl and with a knife slice through meat a few times to cut up smaller.
- Add pepper, salt, and scallions to squash and mix well.
- Create "tot" shapes with your hands and place in air fryer. Spray with olive oil.
- Cook 15 minutes at 350 degrees until golden and crispy!

Cinnamon Butternut Squash Fries

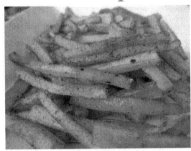

Calories: 175 Fat: 8g Protein: 1g Sugar: 5g
Prep: 10 minutes
Servings: 2

Ingredients:
- 1 pinch of salt
- 1 tbsp. powdered unprocessed sugar
- ½ tsp. nutmeg
- 2 tsp. cinnamon
- 1 tbsp. coconut oil
- 10 ounces pre-cut butternut squash fries

Directions:
- In a plastic bag, pour in all ingredients. Coat fries with other components till coated and sugar is dissolved.
- Spread coated fries into a single layer in the air fryer. Cook 10 minutes at 390 degrees until crispy.

Poultry Recipes

Korean Chicken Wings

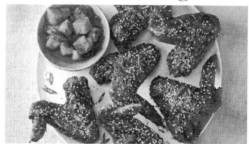

Calories: 356 Fat: 26g Protein: 23g Sugar: 2g
Prep: 10 minutes
Servings: 4

Ingredients:
Wings:
- 1 tsp. pepper
- 1 tsp. salt
- 2 pounds chicken wings

Sauce:
- 2 packets Splenda
- 1 tbsp. minced garlic
- 1 tbsp. minced ginger
- 1 tbsp. sesame oil
- 1 tsp. agave nectar
- 1 tbsp. mayo
- 2 tbsp. gochujang

Finishing:
- ¼ C. chopped green onions
- 2 tsp. sesame seeds

Directions:
- Ensure air fryer is preheated to 400 degrees.

- Line a small pan with foil and place a rack onto the pan, then place into air fryer.
- Season wings with pepper and salt and place onto the rack.
- Air fry 20 minutes, turning at 10 minutes.
- As chicken air fries, mix together all the sauce components.
- Once a thermometer says that the chicken has reached 160 degrees, take out wings and place into a bowl.
- Pour half of the sauce mixture over wings, tossing well to coat.
- Put coated wings back into air fryer for 5 minutes or till they reach 165 degrees.
- Remove and sprinkle with green onions and sesame seeds. Dip into extra sauce.

Buffalo Chicken Wings

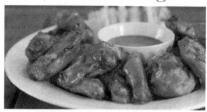

Calories: 402 Fat: 16g Protein: 17g Sugar: 4g
Prep: 15 minutes
Servings: 6-8

Ingredients:

- 1 tsp. salt
- 1-2 tbsp. brown sugar
- 1 tbsp. Worcestershire sauce
- ½ C. vegan butter
- ½ C. cayenne pepper sauce
- 4 pounds chicken wings

Directions:

- Whisk salt, brown sugar, Worcestershire sauce, butter, and hot sauce together and set to the side.
- Dry wings and add to air fryer basket.
- Cook 25 minutes at 380 degrees, tossing halfway through.
- When timer sounds, shake wings and bump up the temperature to 400 degrees and cook another 5 minutes.
- Take out wings and place into a big bowl. Add sauce and toss well.
- Serve alongside celery sticks!

Chicken Fajita Rollups

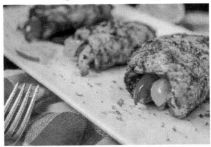

Calories: 189 Fat: 14g Protein: 11g Sugar: 1g
Prep: 5 minutes
Servings: 6-8

Ingredients:

- ½ tsp. oregano
- ½ tsp. cayenne pepper
- 1 tsp. cumin
- 1 tsp. garlic powder
- 2 tsp. paprika
- ½ sliced red onion
- ½ yellow bell pepper, sliced into strips
- ½ green bell pepper, sliced into strips
- ½ red bell pepper, sliced into strips
- 3 chicken breasts

Directions:

- Mix oregano, cayenne pepper, garlic powder, cumin and paprika along with a pinch or two of pepper and salt. Set to the side.
- Slice chicken breasts lengthwise into 2 slices.

- Between two pieces of parchment paper, add breast slices and pound till they are ¼-inch thick. With seasoning, liberally season both sides of chicken slices.
- Put 2 strips of each color of bell pepper and a few onion slices onto chicken pieces.
- Roll up tightly and secure with toothpicks.
- Repeat with remaining ingredients and sprinkle and rub mixture that is left over the chicken rolls.
- Lightly grease your air fryer basket and place 3 rollups into the fryer. Cook 12 minutes at 400 degrees.
- Repeat with remaining rollups.
- Serve with salad!

Crispy Honey Garlic Chicken Wings

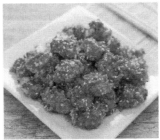

Calories: 435 Fat: 19g Protein: 31g Sugar: 6g
Prep: 15 minutes
Servings: 8

Ingredients:

- 1/8 C. water
- ½ tsp. salt
- 4 tbsp. minced garlic
- ¼ C. vegan butter
- ¼ C. raw honey
- ¾ C. almond flour
- 16 chicken wings

Directions:

- Rinse off and dry chicken wings well. Spray air fryer basket with olive oil.

- Coat chicken wings with almond flour and add coated wings to air fryer. Cook 25 minutes at 380 degrees, shaking every 5 minutes.

- When the timer goes off, cook 5-10 minutes at 400 degrees till skin becomes crispy and dry.

- As chicken cooks, melt butter in a saucepan and add garlic. Sauté garlic 5 minutes. Add salt and honey, simmering 20 minutes. Make sure to stir every so often, so the sauce does not burn. Add a bit of water after 15 minutes to ensure sauce does not harden.

- Take out chicken wings from air fryer and coat in sauce. Enjoy!

Rosemary Turkey Breast with Maple Mustard Glaze

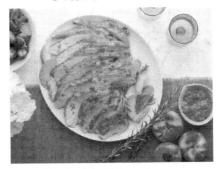

Calories: 278 Fat: 15g Protein: 29g Sugar: 7g
Prep: 15-20 minutes
Servings: 5-7

Ingredients:

- 1 tbsp. vegan butter
- 1 tbsp. stone-ground brown mustard
- ¼ C. pure maple syrup
- 1 tsp. crushed pepper
- 2 tsp. salt
- ½ tsp. dried rosemary
- 2 minced garlic cloves
- ¼ C. olive oil
- 2.5 pounds turkey breast loin

Directions:

- Mix pepper, salt, rosemary, garlic, and olive oil together. Spread herb mixture over turkey breast. Cover and chill 2 hours or overnight to marinade.

- Make sure to remove from fridge about half an hour before cooking.

- Ensure your air fryer is greased well and preheated to 400 degrees. Place loin into the fryer and cook 20 minutes.
- While turkey cooks, melt butter in the microwave. Then add brown mustard and maple syrup.
- Open fryer and spoon on butter mixture over turkey. Cook another 10 minutes.
- Remove turkey from the fryer and let rest 5-10 minutes before attempting to slice.
- Slice against the grain and enjoy!

Mexican Chicken Burgers

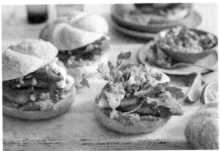

Calories: 234 Fat: 18g Protein: 24g Sugar: 1g
Prep: 5 minutes
Servings: 6-8

Ingredients:
- 1 jalapeno pepper
- 1 tsp. cayenne pepper
- 1 tbsp. mustard powder
- 1 tbsp. oregano
- 1 tbsp. thyme
- 3 tbsp. smoked paprika
- 1 beaten egg
- 1 small head of cauliflower
- 4 chicken breasts

Directions:
- Ensure your air fryer is preheated to 350 degrees.

- Add seasonings to a blender. Slice cauliflower into florets and add to blender.

- Pulse till mixture resembles that of breadcrumbs.

- Take out ¾ of cauliflower mixture and add to a bowl. Set to the side. In another bowl, beat your egg and set to the side.

- Remove skin and bones from chicken breasts and add to blender with remaining cauliflower mixture. Season with pepper and salt.
- Take out mixture and form into burger shapes. Roll each patty in cauliflower crumbs, then the egg, and back into crumbs again.
- Place coated patties into the air fryer, cooking 20 minutes.
- Flip over at 10-minute mark. They are done when crispy!

Crispy Southern Fried Chicken

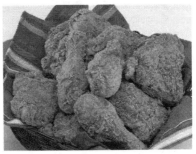

Calories: 504 Fat: 18g Protein: 35g Sugar: 5g
Prep: 10 minutes
Servings: 4

Ingredients:

- 1 tsp. cayenne pepper
- 2 tbsp. mustard powder
- 2 tbsp. oregano
- 2 tbsp. thyme
- 3 tbsp. coconut milk
- 1 beaten egg
- ¼ C. cauliflower
- ¼ C. gluten-free oats
- 8 chicken drumsticks

Directions:

- Ensure air fryer is preheated to 350 degrees.
- Lay out chicken and season with pepper and salt on all sides.

- Add all other ingredients to a blender, blending till a smooth-like breadcrumb mixture is created. Place in a bowl and add a beaten egg to another bowl.
- Dip chicken into breadcrumbs, then into egg, and breadcrumbs once more.
- Place coated drumsticks into air fryer and cook 20 minutes. Bump up the temperature to 390 degrees and cook another 5 minutes till crispy.

Air Fryer Turkey Breast

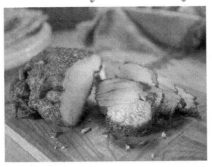

Calories: 212 Fat: 12g Protein: 24g Sugar: 0g
Prep: 5 minutes
Servings: 6-8

Ingredients:

- Pepper and salt
- 1 oven-ready turkey breast
- Turkey seasonings of choice

Directions:

- Preheat air fryer to 350 degrees.
- Season turkey with pepper, salt, and other desired seasonings.
- Place turkey in air fryer basket.
- Cook 60 minutes. The meat should be at 165 degrees when done.
- Allow to rest 10-15 minutes before slicing. Enjoy!

Chicken Kabobs

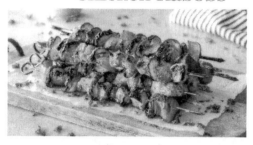

Calories: 296 Fat: 13g Protein: 17g Sugar: 1g
Prep: 15 minutes
Servings: 4

Ingredients:

- 2 diced chicken breasts
- 3 bell peppers
- 6 mushrooms
- Sesame seeds
- 1/3 C. low-sodium soy sauce
- 1/3 C. raw honey

Directions:

- Chop up chicken into cubes, seasoning with a few sprays of olive oil, pepper, and salt.
- Dice up bell peppers and cut mushrooms in half.
- Mix soy sauce and honey together till well combined. Add sesame seeds and stir.
- Skewer chicken, peppers, and mushrooms onto wooden skewers.
- Ensure air fryer is preheated to 388 degrees. Coat kabobs with honey-soy sauce.
- Place coated kabobs in air fryer basket and cook 15-20 minutes.

Mustard Chicken Tenders

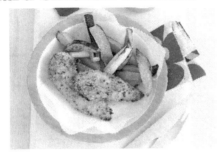

Calories: 403 Fat: 20g Protein: 22g Sugar: 4g
Prep: 10 minutes
Servings: 4-6

Ingredients:

- ½ C. coconut flour
- 1 tbsp. spicy brown mustard
- 2 beaten eggs
- 1 pound of chicken tenders

Directions:

- Season tenders with pepper and salt.

- Place a thin layer of mustard onto tenders and then dredge in flour and dip in egg.

- Add to air fryer and cook 10-15 minutes at 390 degrees till crispy.

Keto Fried "Mock KFC" Chicken

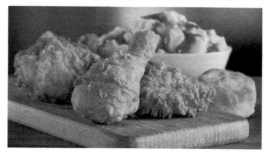

Calories: 521 Fat: 21g Protein: 36g Sugar: 6g
Prep: 15 minutes
Servings: 6

Ingredients:

- 1 tsp. chili flakes
- 1 tsp. curcumin
- 1 tsp. white pepper
- 1 tsp. ginger powder
- 1 tsp. garlic powder
- 1 tsp. paprika
- 1 tsp. powdered mustard
- 1 tsp. pepper
- 1 tbsp. celery salt
- 1/3 tsp. oregano
- ½ tbsp. basil
- ½ tsp. thyme
- 2 garlic cloves
- 1 egg
- 6 boneless, skinless chicken thighs
- 2 tbsp. unsweetened almond milk
- ¼ C. whey protein isolate powder

Directions:

- Wash and pat dry chicken thighs. Slice into small chunks.
- Mash cloves and add them along with all spices in a blender. Blend until smooth and pour over chicken, adding milk and egg. Mix thoroughly.
- Cover chicken and chill for 1 hour.
- Add whey protein to a bowl and dredge coated chicken pieces. Shake excess powder.
- Ensure your air fryer is preheated to 390 degrees. Add coated chicken and cook 20 minutes till crispy, making sure to turn halfway through cooking.

Cheesy Chicken Fritters

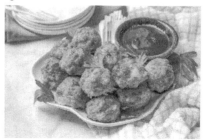

Calories: 467 Fat: 27g Protein: 21g Sugar: 3g
Prep: 10 minutes
Make 16-18 fritters

Ingredients:

Chicken Fritters:
- ½ tsp. salt
- 1/8 tsp. pepper
- 1 ½ tbsp. fresh dill
- 1 1/3 C. shredded mozzarella cheese
- 1/3 C. coconut flour
- 1/3 C. vegan mayo
- 2 eggs
- 1 ½ pounds chicken breasts

Garlic Dip:
- 1/8 tsp. pepper
- ¼ tsp. salt
- ½ tbsp. lemon juice
- 1 pressed garlic cloves
- 1/3 C. vegan mayo

Directions:
- Slice chicken breasts into 1/3" pieces and place in a bowl. Add all remaining fritter ingredients to the bowl and stir well. Cover and chill 2 hours or overnight.

- Ensure your air fryer is preheated to 350 degrees. Spray basket with a bit of olive oil.
- Add marinated chicken to air fryer and cook 20 minutes, making sure to turn halfway through cooking process.
- To make the dipping sauce, combine all the dip ingredients until smooth.

Chinese Salt and Pepper Chicken Wing Stir-Fry

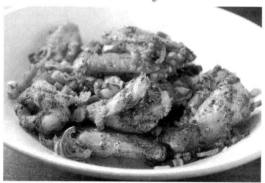

Calories: 351 Fat: 14g Protein: 23g Sugar: 2g
Prep: 15 minutes
Make 14-20 wings

Ingredients:
- ¾ C. potato starch
- ¼ tsp. pepper
- ½ tsp. salt
- 1 egg white
- 14-20 chicken wing pieces

Stir-fry:
- ¼ tsp. pepper
- 1 tsp. sea salt
- 2 tbsp. avocado oil
- 2 trimmed scallions
- 2 jalapeno peppers

Directions:
- Coat air fryer with oil.

- Whisk pepper, salt, and egg white together till foamy.

- Pat wings dry and add to the bowl of egg white mixture.
  Coat well. Let marinate at least 20 minutes.

- Place coated wings in a big bowl and add starch. Dredge wings well. Shake off and add to air fryer basket.
- Cook 25 minutes at 380 degrees. When timer sounds, bump up the temperature to 400 degrees and cook an additional 5 minutes till browned.
- For stir fry, remove seeds from jalapenos and chop up scallions. Add both to bowl and set to the side.
- Heat a wok with oil and add pepper, salt, scallions, and jalapenos. Cook 1 minute. Add air fried chicken to skillet and toss with stir-fried veggies. Cook 60 seconds and devour!

Air Fryer Chicken Parmesan

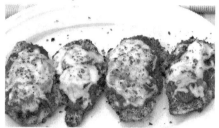

Calories: 251 Fat: 10g Protein: 31g Sugar: 0g
Prep: 15 minutes
Servings: 4
Ingredients:

- ½ C. keto marinara
- 6 tbsp. mozzarella cheese
- 1 tbsp. melted ghee
- 2 tbsp. grated parmesan cheese
- 6 tbsp. gluten-free seasoned breadcrumbs
- 2 8-ounce chicken breasts

Directions:

- Ensure air fryer is preheated to 360 degrees. Spray the basket with olive oil.
- Mix parmesan cheese and breadcrumbs together. Melt ghee.
- Brush melted ghee onto the chicken and dip into breadcrumb mixture.
- Place coated chicken in the air fryer and top with olive oil.
- Cook 2 breasts for 6 minutes and top each breast with a tablespoon of sauce and 1 ½ tablespoons of mozzarella cheese. Cook another 3 minutes to melt cheese.
- Keep cooked pieces warm as you repeat the process with remaining breasts.

Jerk Chicken Wings

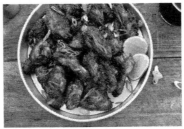

Calories: 374 Fat: 14g Protein: 33g Sugar: 4g
Prep: 10 minutes
Servings: 6-8

Ingredients:

- 1 tsp. salt
- ½ C. red wine vinegar
- 5 tbsp. lime juice
- 4 chopped scallions
- 1 tbsp. grated ginger
- 2 tbsp. brown sugar
- 1 tbsp. chopped thyme
- 1 tsp. white pepper
- 1 tsp. cayenne pepper
- 1 tsp. cinnamon
- 1 tbsp. allspice
- 1 Habanero pepper (seeds/ribs removed and chopped finely)
- 6 chopped garlic cloves
- 2 tbsp. low-sodium soy sauce
- 2 tbsp. olive oil
- 4 pounds of chicken wings

Directions:

- Combine all ingredients except wings in a bowl. Pour into a gallon bag and add chicken wings. Chill 2-24 hours to marinate.

- Ensure your air fryer is preheated to 390 degrees.
- Place chicken wings into a strainer to drain excess liquids.
- Pour half of the wings into your air fryer and cook 14-16 minutes, making sure to shake halfway through the cooking process.
- Remove and repeat the process with remaining wings.

Pork Taquitos

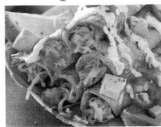

Calories: 309 Fat: 11g Protein: 21g Sugar: 2g
Prep: 10 minutes
Servings: 8

Ingredients:
- 1 juiced lime
- 10 whole wheat tortillas
- 2 ½ C. shredded mozzarella cheese
- 30 ounces of cooked and shredded pork tenderloin

Directions:
- Ensure your air fryer is preheated to 380 degrees.
- Drizzle pork with lime juice and gently mix.
- Heat up tortillas in the microwave with a dampened paper towel to soften.
- Add about 3 ounces of pork and ¼ cup of shredded cheese to each tortilla. Tightly roll them up.
- Spray the air fryer basket with a bit of olive oil.
- Air fry taquitos 7-10 minutes till tortillas turn a slight golden color, making sure to flip halfway through cooking process.

Keto Parmesan Crusted Pork Chops

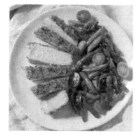

Calories: 422 Fat: 19g Protein: 38g Sugar: 2g
Prep: 10 minutes
Servings: 4-6
Ingredients:

- 3 tbsp. grated parmesan cheese
- 1 C. pork rind crumbs
- 2 beaten eggs
- ¼ tsp. chili powder
- ½ tsp. onion powder
- 1 tsp. smoked paprika
- ¼ tsp. pepper
- ½ tsp. salt
- 4-6 thick boneless pork chops

Directions:

- Ensure your air fryer is preheated to 400 degrees.
- With pepper and salt, season both sides of pork chops.
- In a food processor, pulse pork rinds into crumbs. Mix crumbs with other seasonings.
  Beat eggs and add to another bowl.
- Dip pork chops into eggs then into pork rind crumb mixture.
  Spray down air fryer with olive oil and add pork chops to the basket.
- Cook 12-15 minutes.

Crispy Breaded Pork Chops

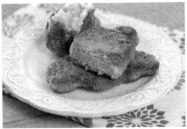

Calories: 378 Fat: 13g Protein: 33g Sugar: 1g
Prep: 15 minutes
Servings: 8

Ingredients:

- 1/8 tsp. pepper
- ¼ tsp. chili powder
- ½ tsp. onion powder
- ½ tsp. garlic powder
- 1 ¼ tsp. sweet paprika
- 2 tbsp. grated parmesan cheese
- 1/3 C. crushed cornflake crumbs
- ½ C. panko breadcrumbs
- 1 beaten egg
- 6 center-cut boneless pork chops

Directions:

- Ensure that your air fryer is preheated to 400 degrees. Spray the basket with olive oil.

- With ½ teaspoon salt and pepper, season both sides of pork chops.

- Combine ¾ teaspoon salt with pepper, chili powder, onion powder, garlic powder, paprika, cornflake crumbs, panko breadcrumbs and parmesan cheese.

- Beat egg in another bowl.
- Dip pork chops into the egg and then crumb mixture.
- Add pork chops to air fryer and spritz with olive oil. Cook 12 minutes, making sure to flip over halfway through cooking process.
- Only add 3 chops in at a time and repeat the process with remaining pork chops.

Chinese Salt and Pepper Pork Chop Stir-fry

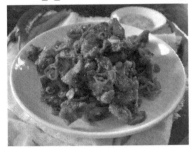

Calories: 294 Fat: 17g Protein: 36g Sugar: 4g
Prep: 10 minutes
Servings: 4

Ingredients:

Pork Chops:
- Olive oil
- ¾ C. almond flour
- ¼ tsp. pepper
- ½ tsp. salt
- 1 egg white
- Pork Chops

Stir-fry:
- ¼ tsp. pepper
- 1 tsp. sea salt
- 2 tbsp. olive oil
- 2 sliced scallions
- 2 sliced jalapeno peppers

Directions:
- Coat the air fryer basket with olive oil.

- Whisk pepper, salt, and egg white together till foamy.

- Cut pork chops into pieces, leaving just a bit on bones.
  Pat dry.

- Add pieces of pork to egg white mixture, coating well. Let sit for marinade 20 minutes.
- Put marinated chops into a large bowl and add almond flour. Dredge and shake off excess and place into air fryer.
- Cook 12 minutes at 360 degrees.
- Turn up the heat to 400 degrees and cook another 6 minutes till pork chops are nice and crisp.
- To make stir-fry, remove jalapeno seeds and chop up. Chop scallions and mix with jalapeno pieces.
- Heat a skillet with olive oil. Stir-fry pepper, salt, scallions, and jalapenos 60 seconds. Then add fried pork pieces to skills and toss with scallion mixture. Stir-fry 1-2 minutes till well coated and hot.

Garlic Putter Pork Chops

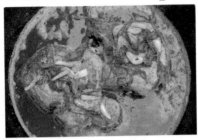

Calories: 526 Fat: 23g Protein: 41g Sugar: 4g
Prep: 5 minutes
Servings: 4

Ingredients:
- 2 tsp. parsley
- 2 tsp. grated garlic cloves
- 1 tbsp. coconut oil
- 1 tbsp. coconut butter
- 4 pork chops

Directions:
- Ensure your air fryer is preheated to 350 degrees.
- Mix butter, coconut oil, and all seasoning together. Then rub seasoning mixture over all sides of pork chops. Place in foil, seal, and chill for 1 hour.
- Remove pork chops from foil and place into air fryer.
- Cook 7 minutes on one side and 8 minutes on the other.
- Drizzle with olive oil and serve alongside a green salad.

Bacon Wrapped Pork Tenderloin

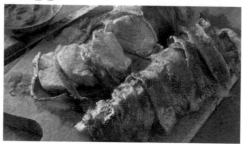

Calories: 554 Fat: 25g Protein: 29g Sugar: 6g
Prep: 10 minutes
Servings: 4-6

Ingredients:
Pork:

- 1-2 tbsp. Dijon mustard
- 3-4 strips of bacon
- 1 pork tenderloin

Apple Gravy:

- ½ - 1 tsp. Dijon mustard
- 1 tbsp. almond flour
- 2 tbsp. ghee
- 1 chopped onion
- 2-3 Granny Smith apples
- 1 C. vegetable broth

Directions:

- Spread Dijon mustard all over tenderloin and wrap meat with strips of bacon.

- Place into air fryer and cook 10-15 minutes at 360 degrees. Use a meat thermometer to check for doneness.

- To make sauce, heat ghee in a pan and add shallots. Cook 1-2 minutes.

- Then add apples, cooking 3-5 minutes until softened. Add flour and ghee to make a roux. Add broth and mustard, stirring well to combine.
- When sauce starts to bubble, add 1 cup of sautéed apples, cooking till sauce thickens.
- Once pork tenderloin I cook, allow to sit 5-10 minutes to rest before slicing.
- Serve topped with apple gravy. Devour!

Dijon Garlic Pork Tenderloin

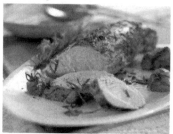

Calories: 423 Fat: 18g Protein: 31g Sugar: 3g
Prep: 5 minutes
Servings: 6-8

Ingredients:
- 1 C. breadcrumbs
- Pinch of cayenne pepper
- 3 crushed garlic cloves
- 2 tbsp. ground ginger
- 2 tbsp. Dijon mustard
- 2 tbsp. raw honey
- 4 tbsp. water
- 2 tsp. salt
- 1 pound pork tenderloin, sliced into 1-inch rounds

Directions:
- With pepper and salt, season all sides of tenderloin.
- Combine cayenne pepper, garlic, ginger, mustard, honey, and water until smooth.
- Dip pork rounds into honey mixture and then into breadcrumbs, ensuring they all get coated well.
- Place coated pork rounds into your air fryer.
- Cook 10 minutes at 400 degrees. Flip and then cook an additional 5 minutes until golden in color.

Cajun Pork Steaks

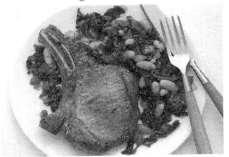

Calories: 209 Fat: 11g Protein: 28g Sugar: 2g
Prep: 5 minutes
Servings: 4-6

Ingredients:
- 4-6 pork steaks

BBQ sauce:
- Cajun seasoning
- 1 tbsp. vinegar
- 1 tsp. low-sodium soy sauce
- ½ C. brown sugar
- ½ C. vegan ketchup

Directions:
- Ensure your air fryer is preheated to 290 degrees.
- Sprinkle pork steaks with Cajun seasoning.
- Combine remaining ingredients and brush onto steaks.
- Add coated steaks to air fryer. Cook 15-20 minutes till just browned.

Air Fryer Sweet and Sour Pork

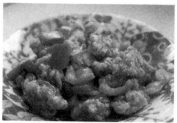

Calories: 371 Fat: 17g Protein: 27g Sugar: 1g
Prep: 15 minutes
Servings: 4-6

Ingredients:

- 3 tbsp. olive oil
- 1/16 tsp. Chinese Five Spice
- ¼ tsp. pepper
- ½ tsp. sea salt
- 1 tsp. pure sesame oil
- 2 eggs
- 1 C. almond flour
- 2 pounds pork, sliced into chunks

Sweet and Sour Sauce:

- ¼ tsp. sea salt
- ½ tsp. garlic powder
- 1 tbsp. low-sodium soy sauce
- ½ C. rice vinegar
- 5 tbsp. tomato paste
- 1/8 tsp. water
- ½ C. sweetener of choice

Directions:

- To make the dipping sauce, whisk all sauce ingredients together over medium heat, stirring 5 minutes. Simmer uncovered 5 minutes till thickened.

- Meanwhile, combine almond flour, five spice, pepper, and salt.
- In another bowl, mix eggs with sesame oil.
- Dredge pork in flour mixture and then in egg mixture. Shake any excess off before adding to air fryer basket.
- Cook 8-12 minutes at 340 degrees.
- Serve with sweet and sour dipping sauce!

Roasted Char Siew (Pork Butt)

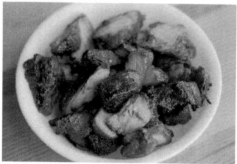

Calories: 289 Fat: 13g Protein: 33g Sugar: 1g
Prep: 15 minutes
Servings: 4-6

Ingredients:

- 1 strip of pork shoulder butt with a good amount of fat marbling

Marinade:

- 1 tsp. sesame oil
- 4 tbsp. raw honey
- 1 tsp. low-sodium dark soy sauce
- 1 tsp. light soy sauce
- 1 tbsp. rose wine
- 2 tbsp. Hoisin sauce

Directions:

- Combine all marinade ingredients together and add to Ziploc bag. Place pork in bag, making sure all sections of pork strip are engulfed in the marinade. Chill 3-24 hours.

- Take out the strip 30 minutes before planning to cook and preheat your air fryer to 350 degrees.

- Place foil on small pan and brush with olive oil. Place marinated pork strip onto prepared pan.
- Roast 20 minutes.
- Glaze with marinade every 5-10 minutes.
- Remove strip and leave to cool a few minutes before slicing.

Roasted Pork Loin

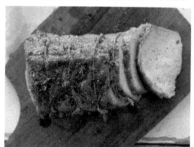

Calories: 511 Fat: 18g Protein: 43g Sugar: 1g
Prep: 10 minutes
Servings: 6-8

Ingredients:

- Balsamic vinegar
- 1 tsp. parsley
- ½ tsp. red pepper flakes
- ½ tsp. garlic powder
- 1 tsp. pepper
- 1 tsp. sat
- 2-pound pork loin

Directions:

- Sprinkle pork loin with seasonings and brush with vinegar.
- Place pork in your air fryer. Cook 25 minutes at 340 degrees.
- Remove from air fryer and let rest 10 minutes before slicing.

Teriyaki Pork Rolls

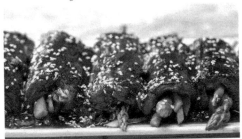

Calories: 412 Fat: 9g Protein: 19g Sugar: 4g
Prep: 5 minutes
Servings: 4-8

Ingredients:
- 1 tsp. almond flour
- 4 tbsp. low-sodium soy sauce
- 4 tbsp. mirin
- 4 tbsp. brown sugar
- Thumb-sized amount of ginger, chopped
- Pork belly slices
- Enoki mushrooms

Directions:
- Mix brown sugar, mirin, soy sauce, almond flour, and ginger together until brown sugar dissolves.
- Take pork belly slices and wrap around a bundle of mushrooms. Brush each roll with teriyaki sauce. Chill half an hour.
- Preheat your air fryer to 350 degrees and add marinated pork rolls.
- Cook 8 minutes.

Ham and Cheese Rollups

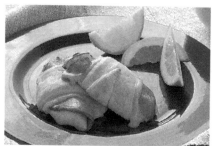

Calories: 289 Fat: 6g Protein: 18g Sugar: 4g
Prep: 2 minutes
Servings: 12

Ingredients:

- 2 tsp. raw honey
- 2 tsp. dried parsley
- 1 tbsp. poppy seeds
- ½ C. melted coconut oil
- ¼ C. spicy brown mustard
- 9 slices of provolone cheese
- 10 ounces of thinly sliced Black Forest Ham
- 1 tube of crescent rolls

Directions:

- Roll out dough into a rectangle. Spread 2-3 tablespoons of spicy mustard onto dough, then layer provolone cheese and ham slices.

- Roll the filled dough up as tight as you can and slice into 12-15 pieces.

- Melt coconut oil and mix with a pinch of salt and pepper, parsley, honey, and remaining mustard.

- Brush mustard mixture over roll-ups and sprinkle with poppy seeds.
- Grease air fryer basket liberally with olive oil and add rollups.
- Cook 15 minutes at 350 degrees.
- Serve!

New York Style Pork Egg Rolls

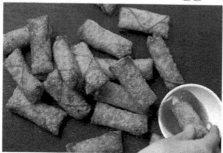

Calories: 578 Fat: 11g Protein: 14g Sugar: 4g
Prep: 10 minutes
Makes 12 egg rolls

Ingredients:

- 1 C. sweet and sour sauce recipe (from the previous recipe)
- 1 C. olive oil
- 1 egg
- 12 egg roll wrappers
- 4 C. pressure cooker egg roll recipe

Directions:

- Mix up the sweet and sour sauce.

- Crack egg and whisk.

- Lay out egg roll wrappers, with corners facing to you. Moisten the edges with egg wash.

- Take 1/3 of a cup of egg roll filling and place into wrappers.

- Fold the bottom point over filling and tuck underneath filling. Fold both sides, ensuring they stick to the first flap you made. Roll it up tightly and seal with more egg wash. Repeat till you use all ingredients.

- Place egg rolls into air fryer basket. Spray with olive oil.
- Cook 10 minutes at 390 degrees, making sure you turn halfway through the cooking process.
- Serve with sweet and sour dipping sauce!

Vietnamese Pork Chops

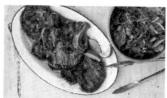

Calories: 290 Fat: 15g Protein: 30g Sugar: 3g
Prep: 10 minutes
Servings: 2

Ingredients:
- 1 tbsp. olive oil
- 1 tbsp. fish sauce
- 1 tsp. low-sodium dark soy sauce
- 1 tsp. pepper
- 3 tbsp. lemongrass
- 1 tbsp. chopped shallot
- 1 tbsp. chopped garlic
- 1 tbsp. brown sugar
- 2 pork chops

Directions:
- Add pork chops to a bowl along with olive oil, fish sauce, soy sauce, pepper, lemongrass, shallot, garlic, and brown sugar.
- Marinade pork chops 2 hours.
- Ensure your air fryer is preheated to 400 degrees. Add pork chops to the basket.
- Cook 7 minutes, making sure to flip after 5 minutes of cooking.
- Serve alongside steamed cauliflower rice!

Beef Recipes

Cheeseburger Egg Rolls

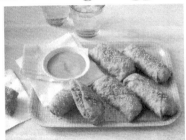

Calories: 153 Fat: 4g Protein: 12g Sugar: 3g
Prep: 15 minutes
Makes 6 egg rolls

Ingredients:
- 6 egg roll wrappers
- 6 chopped dill pickle chips
- 1 tbsp. yellow mustard
- 3 tbsp. cream cheese
- 3 tbsp. shredded cheddar cheese
- ½ C. chopped onion
- ½ C. chopped bell pepper
- ¼ tsp. onion powder
- ¼ tsp. garlic powder
- 8 ounces of raw lean ground beef

Directions:
- In a skillet, add seasonings, beef, onion, and bell pepper. Stir and crumble beef till fully cooked, and vegetables are soft.
- Take skillet off the heat and add cream cheese, mustard, and cheddar cheese, stirring till melted.

- Pour beef mixture into a bowl and fold in pickles.
- Lay out egg wrappers and place 1/6th of beef mixture into each one. Moisten egg roll wrapper edges with water. Fold sides to the middle and seal with water.
- Repeat with all other egg rolls.
- Place rolls into air fryer, one batch at a time. Cook 7-9 minutes at 392 degrees.

Copycat Taco Bell Crunch Wraps

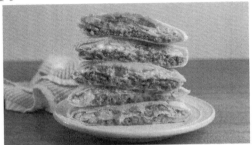

Calories: 311 Fat: 9g Protein: 22g Sugar: 2g
Prep: 5 minutes
Servings: 6

Ingredients:

- 6 wheat tostadas
- 2 C. sour cream
- 2 C. Mexican blend cheese
- 2 C. shredded lettuce
- 12 ounces low-sodium nacho cheese
- 3 Roma tomatoes
- 6 12-inch wheat tortillas
- 1 1/3 C. water
- 2 packets low-sodium taco seasoning
- 2 pounds of lean ground beef

Directions:

- Ensure your air fryer is preheated to 400 degrees.

- Make beef according to taco seasoning packets.

- Place 2/3 C. prepared beef, 4 tbsp. cheese, 1 tostada, 1/3 C. sour cream, 1/3 C. lettuce, 1/6th of tomatoes and 1/3 C. cheese on each tortilla.

- Fold up tortillas edges and repeat with remaining ingredients.

Lay the folded sides of tortillas down into the air fryer and spray with olive oil.

- Cook 2 minutes till browned.

Country Fried Steak

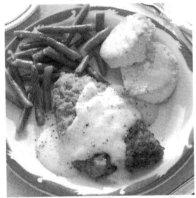

Calories: 395 Fat: 11g Protein: 39g Sugar: 5g
Prep: 10 minutes
Servings: 2

Ingredients:

- 1 tsp. pepper
- 2 C. almond milk
- 2 tbsp. almond flour
- 6 ounces ground sausage meat
- 1 tsp. pepper
- 1 tsp. salt
- 1 tsp. garlic powder
- 1 tsp. onion powder
- 1 C. panko breadcrumbs
- 1 C. almond flour
- 3 beaten eggs
- 6 ounces sirloin steak, pounded till thin

Directions:

- Season panko breadcrumbs with spices. Dredge steak in flour, then egg, and then seasoned panko mixture.

- Place into air fryer basket. Cook 12 minutes at 370 degrees.
- To make sausage gravy, cook sausage and drain off fat, but reserve 2 tablespoons.
- Add flour to sausage and mix until incorporated. Gradually mix in milk over medium to high heat till it becomes thick.
- Season mixture with pepper and cook 3 minutes longer.
- Serve steak topped with gravy and enjoy!

Air Fryer Roast Beef

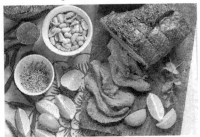

Calories: 267 Fat: 8g Protein: 21g Sugar: 1g
Prep: 10 minutes
Servings: 6-8

Ingredients:
- Roast beef
- 1 tbsp. olive oil
- Seasonings of choice

Directions:
- Ensure your air fryer is preheated to 160 degrees.
- Place roast in bowl and toss with olive oil and desired seasonings.
- Put seasoned roast into air fryer and cook 30 minutes.
- Turn roast when the timer sounds and cook another 15 minutes.

Crispy Mongolian Beef

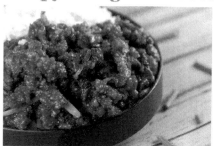

Calories: 290 Fat: 14g Protein: 22g Sugar: 1g
Prep: 10 minutes
Servings: 6-10

Ingredients:
- Olive oil
- ½ C. almond flour
- 2 pounds beef tenderloin or beef chuck, sliced into strips

Sauce:
- ½ C. chopped green onion
- 1 tsp. red chili flakes
- 1 tsp. almond flour
- ½ C. brown sugar
- 1 tsp. hoisin sauce
- ½ C. water
- ½ C. rice vinegar
- ½ C. low-sodium soy sauce
- 1 tbsp. chopped garlic
- 1 tbsp. finely chopped ginger
- 2 tbsp. olive oil

Directions:
- Toss strips of beef in almond flour, ensuring they are coated well.

- Add to air fryer and cook 10 minutes at 300 degrees.

- Meanwhile, add all sauce ingredients to the pan and bring to a boil. Mix well.
- Add beef strips to the sauce and cook 2 minutes.
- Serve over cauliflower rice!

Beef Taco Fried Egg Rolls

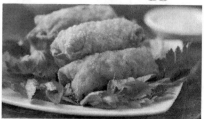

Calories: 348 Fat: 11g Protein: 24g Sugar: 1g
Prep: 15 minutes
Makes 8 egg rolls

Ingredients:

- 1 tsp. cilantro
- 2 chopped garlic cloves
- 1 tbsp. olive oil
- 1 C. shredded Mexican cheese
- ½ packet taco seasoning
- ½ can cilantro lime rotel
- ½ chopped onion
- 16 egg roll wrappers
- 1 pound lean ground beef

Directions:

- Ensure that your air fryer is preheated to 400 degrees.

- Add onions and garlic to a skillet, cooking till fragrant. Then add taco seasoning, pepper, salt, and beef, cooking till beef is broke up into tiny pieces and cooked thoroughly.

- Add rotel and stir well.

- Lay out egg wrappers and brush with water to soften a bit.

- Load wrappers with beef filling and add cheese to each.

- Fold diagonally to close and use water to secure edges.
- Brush filled egg wrappers with olive oil and add to the air fryer.
- Cook 8 minutes, flip, and cook another 4 minutes.
- Served sprinkled with cilantro.

Pub Style Corned Beef Egg Rolls

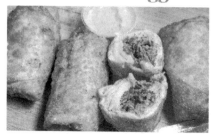

Calories: 415 Fat: 13g Protein: 38g Sugar: 4g
Prep: 5 minutes
Makes 10 egg rolls

Ingredients:
- Olive oil
- ½ C. orange marmalade
- 5 slices of Swiss cheese
- 4 C. corned beef and cabbage
- 1 egg
- 10 egg roll wrappers

Brandy Mustard Sauce:
- 1/16th tsp. pepper
- 2 tbsp. whole grain mustard
- 1 tsp. dry mustard powder
- 1 C. heavy cream
- ½ C. chicken stock
- ¼ C. brandy
- ¾ C. dry white wine
- ¼ tsp. curry powder
- ½ tbsp. cilantro
- 1 minced shallot
- 2 tbsp. ghee

Directions:
- To make mustard sauce, add shallots and ghee to skillet, cooking until softened. Then add brandy and wine, heating to a low boil. Cook 5 minutes for liquids

to reduce. Add stock and seasonings. Simmer 5 minutes.

- Turn down heat and add heavy cream. Cook on low till sauce reduces and it covers the back of a spoon.
- Place sauce in the fridge to chill.
- Crack the egg in a bowl and set to the side.
- Lay out an egg wrapper with the corner towards you. Brush the edges with egg wash.
- Place 1/3 cup of corned beef mixture into the center along with 2 tablespoons of marmalade and ½ a slice of Swiss cheese.
- Fold the bottom corner over filling. As you are folding the sides, make sure they are stick well to the first flap you made.
- Place filled rolls into prepared air fryer basket. Spritz rolls with olive oil.
- Cook 10 minutes at 390 degrees, shaking halfway through cooking.
- Serve rolls with Brandy Mustard sauce and devour!

Reuben Egg Rolls

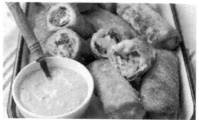

Calories: 251 Fat: 12g Protein: 31g Sugar: 4g
Prep: 5 minutes
Makes 4-6 egg rolls

Ingredients:
- Swiss cheese
- Can of sauerkraut
- Sliced deli corned beef
- Egg roll wrappers

Directions:
- Cut corned beef and Swiss cheese into thin slices.

- Drain sauerkraut and dry well.

- Take egg roll wrapper and moisten edges with water.

- Stack center with corned beef and cheese till you reach desired thickness. Top off with sauerkraut.

- Fold corner closest to you over the edge of filling. Bring up sides and glue with water.

- Add to air fryer basket and spritz with olive oil.

- Cook 4 minutes at 400 degrees, then flip and cook another 4 minutes.

Herbed Roast Beef

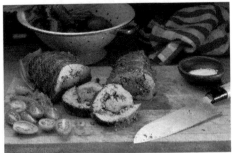

Calories: 502 Fat: 18g Protein: 48g Sugar: 2g
Prep: 15 minutes
Servings: 10-12

Ingredients:
- ½ tsp. fresh rosemary
- 1 tsp. dried thyme
- ¼ tsp. pepper
- 1 tsp. salt
- 4-pound top round roast beef
- 2 tsp. olive oil

Directions:
- Ensure your air fryer is preheated to 360 degrees.

- Rub olive oil all over beef.

- Mix rosemary, thyme, pepper, and salt together and proceed to rub all sides of beef with spice mixture.

- Place seasoned beef into air fryer and cook 20 minutes.

- Allow roast to rest 10 minutes before slicing to serve.

Beef Empanadas

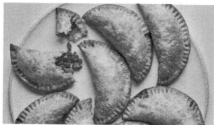

Calories: 183 Fat: 5g Protein: 11g Sugar: 2g
Prep: 15 minutes
Servings: 8

Ingredients:

- 1 tsp. water
- 1 egg white
- 1 C. picadillo
- 8 Goya empanada discs (thawed)

Directions:

- Ensure your air fryer is preheated to 325. Spray basket with olive oil.

- Place 2 tablespoons of picadillo into the center of each disc. Fold disc in half and use a fork to seal edges. Repeat with all ingredients.

- Whisk egg white with water and brush tops of empanadas with egg wash.

- Add 2-3 empanadas to air fryer, cooking 8 minutes until golden. Repeat till you cook all filled empanadas.

Air Fryer Burgers

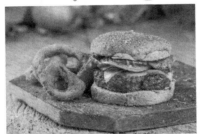

Calories: 148 Fat: 5g Protein: 24g Sugar: 1g
Prep: 10 minutes
Servings: 4

Ingredients:
- 1 pound lean ground beef
- 1 tsp. dried parsley
- ½ tsp. dried oregano
- ½ tsp. pepper
- ½ tsp. salt
- ½ tsp. onion powder
- ½ tsp. garlic powder
- Few drops of liquid smoke
- 1 tsp. Worcestershire sauce

Directions:
- Ensure your air fryer is preheated to 350 degrees.

- Mix all seasonings together till combined.

- Place beef in a bowl and add seasonings. Mix well, but do not overmix.

- Make 4 patties from the mixture and using your thumb, making an indent in the center of each patty.

- Add patties to air fryer basket and cook 10 minutes. No need to turn!

Roasted Stuffed Peppers

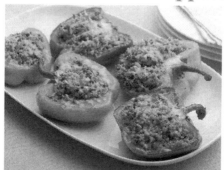

Calories: 295 Fat: 8g Protein: 23g Sugar: 2g
Prep: 5 minutes
Servings: 4

Ingredients:

- 4 ounces shredded cheddar cheese
- ½ tsp. pepper
- ½ tsp. salt
- 1 tsp. Worcestershire sauce
- ½ C. tomato sauce
- 8 ounces lean ground beef
- 1 tsp. olive oil
- 1 minced garlic clove
- ½ chopped onion
- 2 green peppers

Directions:

- Ensure your air fryer is preheated to 390 degrees. Spray with olive oil.

- Cut stems off bell peppers and remove seeds. Cook in boiling salted water for 3 minutes.

- Sauté garlic and onion together in a skillet until golden in color.

- Take skillet off the heat. Mix pepper, salt, Worcestershire sauce, ¼ cup of tomato sauce, half of cheese and beef together.
- Divide meat mixture into pepper halves. Top filled peppers with remaining cheese and tomato sauce.
- Place filled peppers in air fryer and bake 15-20 minutes.

Air Fryer Beef Steak

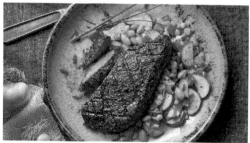

Calories: 233 Fat: 19g Protein: 16g Sugar: 0g
Prep: 17 minutes
Servings: 4

Ingredients:
- 1 tbsp. olive oil
- Pepper and salt
- 2 pounds of ribeye steak

Directions:
- Season meat on both sides with pepper and salt.

- Rub all sides of meat with olive oil.

- Preheat air fryer to 356 degrees and spritz with olive oil.

- Cook steak 7 minutes. Flip and cook an additional 6 minutes.

- Let meat sit 2-5 minutes to rest. Slice and serve with salad.

Beef and Broccoli

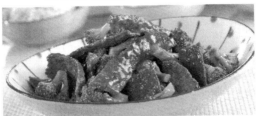

Calories: 384 Fat: 16g Protein: 19g Sugar: 4g
Prep: 10 minutes
Servings: 4

Ingredients:
- 1 minced garlic clove
- 1 sliced ginger root
- 1 tbsp. olive oil
- 1 tsp. almond flour
- 1 tsp. sweetener of choice
- 1 tsp. low-sodium soy sauce
- 1/3 C. sherry
- 2 tsp. sesame oil
- 1/3 C. oyster sauce
- 1 pounds of broccoli
- ¾ pound round steak

Directions:
- Remove stems from broccoli and slice into florets. Slice steak into thin strips.

- Combine sweetener, soy sauce, sherry, almond flour, sesame oil, and oyster sauce together, stirring till sweetener dissolves.

- Put strips of steak into the mixture and allow to marinate 45 minutes to 2 hours.

- Add broccoli and marinated steak to air fryer. Place garlic, ginger, and olive oil on top.
- Cook 12 minutes at 400 degrees. Serve with cauliflower rice!

Air Fryer Beef Fajitas

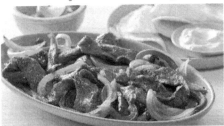

Calories: 412 Fat: 21g Protein: 13g Sugar: 1g
Prep: 5 minutes
Servings: 4-6

Ingredients:
Beef:
- 1/8 C. carne asada seasoning
- 2 pounds beef flap meat
- Diet 7-Up

Fajita veggies:
- 1 tsp. chili powder
- 1-2 tsp. pepper
- 1-2 tsp. salt
- 2 bell peppers, your choice of color
- 1 onion

Directions:
- Slice flap meat into manageable pieces and place into a bowl. Season meat with carne seasoning and pour diet soda over meat. Cover and chill overnight.

- Ensure your air fryer is preheated to 380 degrees.

- Place a parchment liner into air fryer basket and spray with olive oil. Place beef in layers into the basket.

- Cook 8-10 minutes, making sure to flip halfway through. Remove and set to the side.

- Slice up veggies and spray air fryer basket. Add veggies to the fryer and spray with olive oil. Cook 10 minutes at 400 degrees, shaking 1-2 times during cooking process.
- Serve meat and veggies on wheat tortillas and top with favorite keto fillings!

Seafood Recipes

Coconut Shrimp

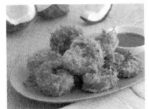

Calories: 213 Fat: 8g Protein: 15g Sugar: 3g
Prep: 5 minutes
Servings: 3
Ingredients:

- 1 C. almond flour
- 1 C. panko breadcrumbs
- 1 tbsp. coconut flour
- 1 C. unsweetened, dried coconut
- 1 egg white
- 12 raw large shrimp

Directions:

- Put shrimp on paper towels to drain.

- Mix coconut and panko breadcrumbs together. Then mix in coconut flour and almond flour in a different bowl. Set to the side.

- Dip shrimp into flour mixture, then into egg white, and then into coconut mixture.

- Place into air fryer basket. Repeat with remaining shrimp.

- Cook 10 minutes at 350 degrees. Turn halfway through cooking process.

Air Fryer Salmon

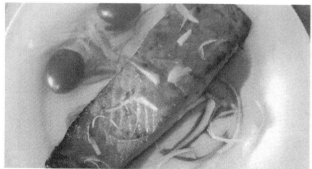

Calories: 185 Fat: 11g Protein: 21g Sugar: 0g
Prep: 5 minutes
Servings: 2

Ingredients:

- ½ tsp. salt
- ½ tsp. garlic powder
- ½ tsp. smoked paprika
- Salmon

Directions:

- Mix spices together and sprinkle onto salmon.

- Place seasoned salmon into air fryer.

- Cook 8-10 minutes at 400 degrees.

Healthy Fish and Chips

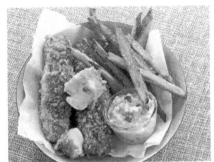

Calories: 219 Carbs: 18 Fat: 5g Protein: 25g Sugar: 1g
Prep: 15 minutes
Servings: 3

Ingredients:

- Old Bay seasoning
- ½ C. panko breadcrumbs
- 1 egg
- 2 tbsp. almond flour
- 2 4-6 ounce tilapia fillets
- Frozen crinkle cut fries

Directions:

- Add almond flour to one bowl, beat egg in another bowl, and add panko breadcrumbs to the third bowl, mixed with Old Bay seasoning.

- Dredge tilapia in flour, then egg, and then breadcrumbs.

- Place coated fish in air fryer along with fries.

- Cook 15 minutes at 390 degrees.

3-Ingredient Air Fryer Catfish

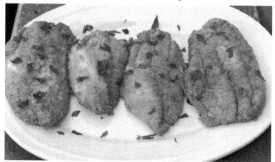

Calories: 208 Carbs: 8 Fat: 5g Protein: 17g Sugar: 0.5g
Prep: 15 minutes
Servings: 4

Ingredients:
- 1 tbsp. chopped parsley
- 1 tbsp. olive oil
- ¼ C. seasoned fish fry
- 4 catfish fillets

Directions:
- Ensure your air fryer is preheated to 400 degrees.

- Rinse off catfish fillets and pat dry.

- Add fish fry seasoning to Ziploc baggie, then catfish. Shake bag and ensure fish gets well coated.

- Spray each fillet with olive oil.

- Add fillets to air fryer basket. Cook 10 minutes. Then flip and cook another 2-3 minutes.

Bang Bang Panko Breaded Fried Shrimp

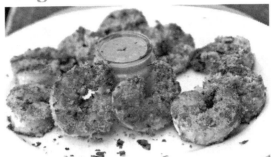

Calories: 212 Carbs: 12 Fat: 1g Protein: 37g Sugar: 0.5g
Prep: 15 minutes
Servings: 4

Ingredients:

- 1 tsp. paprika
- Montreal chicken seasoning
- ¾ C. panko bread crumbs
- ½ C. almond flour
- 1 egg white
- 1 pound raw shrimp (peeled and deveined)

Bang Bang Sauce:

- ¼ C. sweet chili sauce
- 2 tbsp. sriracha sauce
- 1/3 C. plain Greek yogurt

Directions:

- Ensure your air fryer is preheated to 400 degrees. Season all shrimp with seasonings.

- Add flour to one bowl, egg white in another, and breadcrumbs to a third.

- Dip seasoned shrimp in flour, then egg whites, and then breadcrumbs.

- Spray coated shrimp with olive oil and add to air fryer basket.
- Cook 4 minutes, flip, and cook an additional 4 minutes.
- To make the sauce, mix together all sauce ingredients until smooth.

Louisiana Shrimp Po Boy

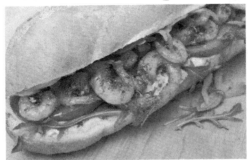

Calories: 337 Carbs: 55 Fat: 12g Protein: 24g Sugar: 2g
Prep: 15 minutes
Servings: 4

Ingredients:

- 1 tsp. creole seasoning
- 8 slices of tomato
- Lettuce leaves
- ¼ C. buttermilk
- ½ C. Louisiana Fish Fry
- 1 pound deveined shrimp

Remoulade sauce:

- 1 chopped green onion
- 1 tsp. hot sauce
- 1 tsp. Dijon mustard
- ½ tsp. creole seasoning
- 1 tsp. Worcestershire sauce
- Juice of ½ a lemon
- ½ C. vegan mayo

Directions:

- To make the sauce, combine all sauce ingredients until well incorporated. Chill while you cook shrimp.

- Mix seasonings together and liberally season shrimp.
- Add buttermilk to a bowl. Dip each shrimp into milk and place in a Ziploc bag. Chill half an hour to marinate.
- Add fish fry to a bowl. Take shrimp from marinating bag and dip into fish fry, then add to air fryer.
- Ensure your air fryer is preheated to 400 degrees.
- Spray shrimp with olive oil. Cook 5 minutes, flip and then cook another 5 minutes.
- Assemble "Keto" Po Boy by adding sauce to lettuce leaves, along with shrimp and tomato.

Air Fryer Salmon Patties

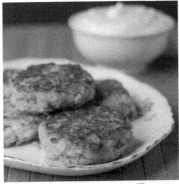

Calories: 437 Carbs: 55 Fat: 12g Protein: 24g Sugar: 2g
Prep: 15 minutes
Servings: 4

Ingredients:

- 1 tbsp. olive oil
- 1 tbsp. ghee
- ¼ tsp. salt
- 1/8 tsp. pepper
- 1 egg
- 1 C. almond flour
- 1 can wild Alaskan pink salmon

Directions:

- Drain can of salmon into a bowl and keep liquid. Discard skin and bones.
- Add salt, pepper, and egg to salmon, mixing well with hands to incorporate. Make patties.
- Dredge in flour and remaining egg. If it seems dry, spoon reserved salmon liquid from the can onto patties.
- Add patties to air fryer. Cook 7 minutes at 378 degrees till golden, making sure to flip once during cooking process.

Fried Calamari

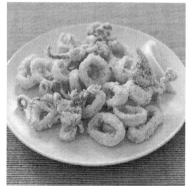

Calories: 211 Fat: 6g Protein: 21g Sugar: 1g
Prep: 15 minutes
Servings: 6-8

Ingredients:

- ½ tsp. salt
- ½ tsp. Old Bay seasoning
- 1/3 C. plain cornmeal
- ½ C. semolina flour
- ½ C. almond flour
- 5-6 C. olive oil
- 1 ½ pounds baby squid

Directions:

- Rinse squid in cold water and slice tentacles, keeping just ¼-inch of the hood in one piece.
- Combine 1-2 pinches of pepper, salt, Old Bay seasoning, cornmeal, and both flours together. Dredge squid pieces into flour mixture and place into air fryer. Spray liberally with olive oil.
- Cook 15 minutes at 345 degrees till coating turns a golden brown.

Panko-Crusted Tilapia

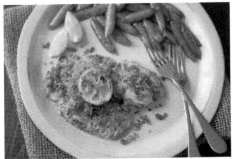

Calories: 256 Fat: 9g Protein: 39g Sugar: 5g
Prep: 5 minutes
Servings: 3

Ingredients:

- 2 tsp. Italian seasoning
- 2 tsp. lemon pepper
- 1/3 C. panko breadcrumbs
- 1/3 C. egg whites
- 1/3 C. almond flour
- 3 tilapia fillets
- Olive oil

Directions:

- Place panko, egg whites, and flour into separate bowls. Mix lemon pepper and Italian seasoning in with breadcrumbs.
- Pat tilapia fillets dry. Dredge in flour, then egg, then breadcrumb mixture. Add to air fryer basket and spray lightly with olive oil.
- Cook 10-11 minutes at 400 degrees, making sure to flip halfway through cooking.

Salmon Croquettes

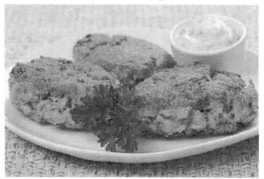

Calories: 503 Carbs: 61g Fat: 9g Protein: 5g Sugar: 4g
Prep: 15 minutes
Servings: 6-8

Ingredients:
- Panko breadcrumbs
- Almond flour
- 2 egg whites
- 2 tbsp. chopped chives
- 2 tbsp. minced garlic cloves
- ½ C. chopped onion
- 2/3 C. grated carrots
- 1 pound chopped salmon fillet

Directions:
- Mix together all ingredients minus breadcrumbs, flour, and egg whites.
- Shape mixture into balls. Then coat them in flour, then egg, and then breadcrumbs. Drizzle with olive oil.
- Add coated salmon balls to air fryer and cook 6 minutes at 350 degrees. Shake and cook an additional 4 minutes until golden in color.

Air Fryer Fish Tacos

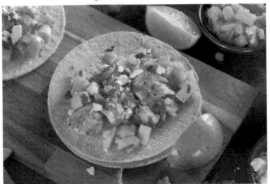

Calories: 178 Fat: 10g Protein: 19g Sugar: 1g
Prep: 5 minutes
Servings: 4

Ingredients:

- 1 pound cod
- 1 tbsp. cumin
- ½ tbsp. chili powder
- 1 ½ C. almond flour
- 1 ½ C. coconut flour
- 10 ounces Mexican beer
- 2 eggs

Directions:

- Whisk beer and eggs together.
- Whisk flours, pepper, salt, cumin, and chili powder together.
  Slice cod into large pieces and coat in egg mixture then flour mixture.
- Spray bottom of your air fryer basket with olive oil and add coated codpieces.
- Cook 15 minutes at 375 degrees.
- Serve on lettuce leaves topped with homemade salsa!

Bacon Wrapped Scallops

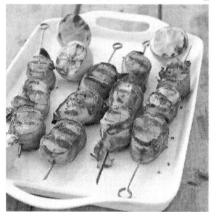

Calories: 389 Fat: 17g Protein: 21g Sugar: 1g
Prep: 10 minutes
Servings: 4

Ingredients:
- 1 tsp. paprika
- 1 tsp. lemon pepper
- 5 slices of center-cut bacon
- 20 raw sea scallops

Directions:
- Rinse and drain scallops, placing on paper towels to soak up excess moisture.
- Cut slices of bacon into 4 pieces.
- Wrap each scallop with a piece of bacon, using toothpicks to secure. Sprinkle wrapped scallops with paprika and lemon pepper.
- Spray air fryer basket with olive oil and add scallops.
- Cook 5-6 minutes at 400 degrees, making sure to flip halfway through.

Parmesan Shrimp

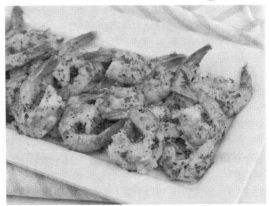

Calories: 351 Fat: 11g Protein: 19g Sugar: 1g
Prep: 10 minutes
Servings: 4-6

Ingredients:

- 2 tbsp. olive oil
- 1 tsp. onion powder
- 1 tsp. basil
- ½ tsp. oregano
- 1 tsp. pepper
- 2/3 C. grated parmesan cheese
- 4 minced garlic cloves
- 2 pounds of jumbo cooked shrimp (peeled/deveined)

Directions:

- Mix all seasonings together and gently toss shrimp with mixture.
- Spray olive oil into air fryer basket and add seasoned shrimp.
- Cook 8-10 minutes at 350 degrees.
- Squeeze lemon juice over shrimp right before devouring!

Honey Glazed Salmon

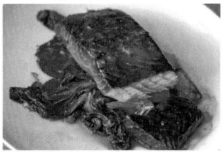

Calories: 390 Fat: 8g Protein: 16g Sugar: 5g
Prep: 5 minutes
Servings: 2
Ingredients:

- 1 tsp. water
- 3 tsp. rice wine vinegar
- 6 tbsp. low-sodium soy sauce
- 6 tbsp. raw honey
- 2 salmon fillets

Directions:

- Combine water, vinegar, honey, and soy sauce together. Pour half of this mixture into a bowl.
- Place salmon in one bowl of marinade and let chill 2 hours.
- Ensure your air fryer is preheated to 356 degrees and add salmon.
- Cook 8 minutes, flipping halfway through. Baste salmon with some of the remaining marinade mixture and cook another 5 minutes.
- To make a sauce to serve salmon with, pour remaining marinade mixture into a saucepan, heating till simmering. Let simmer 2 minutes. Serve drizzled over salmon!

Crispy Air Fried Sushi Roll

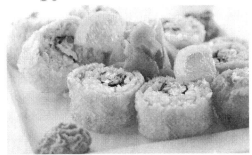

Calories: 267 Fat: 13g Protein: 6g Sugar: 3g
Prep: 15 minutes
Servings: 12

Ingredients:
Kale Salad:
- 1 tbsp. sesame seeds
- ¾ tsp. soy sauce
- ¼ tsp. ginger
- 1/8 tsp. garlic powder
- ¾ tsp. toasted sesame oil
- ½ tsp. rice vinegar
- 1 ½ C. chopped kale

Sushi Rolls:
- ½ of a sliced avocado
- 3 sheets of sushi nori
- 1 batch cauliflower rice

Sriracha Mayo:
- Sriracha sauce
- ¼ C. vegan mayo

Coating:
- ½ C. panko breadcrumbs

Directions:
- Combine all of kale salad ingredients together, tossing well. Set to the side.

- Lay out a sheet of nori and spread a handful of rice on. Then place 2-3 tbsp. of kale salad over rice, followed by avocado. Roll up sushi.
- To make mayo, whisk mayo ingredients together until smooth.
- Add breadcrumbs to a bowl. Coat sushi rolls in crumbs till coated and add to air fryer.
- Cook rolls 10 minutes at 390 degrees, shaking gently at 5 minutes.
- Slice each roll into 6-8 pieces and enjoy!

Sweet Recipes

Perfect Cinnamon Toast

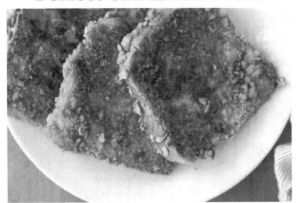

Calories: 124 Fat: 2g Protein: 0g Sugar: 4g
Prep: 5 minutes
Servings: 6
Ingredients:

- 2 tsp. pepper
- 1 ½ tsp. vanilla extract
- 1 ½ tsp. cinnamon
- ½ C. sweetener of choice
- 1 C. coconut oil
- 12 slices whole wheat bread

Directions:

- Melt coconut oil and mix with sweetener until dissolved. Mix in remaining ingredients minus bread till incorporated.
- Spread mixture onto bread, covering all area. Place coated pieces of bread in your air fryer.
- Cook 5 minutes at 400 degrees.
- Remove and cut diagonally. Enjoy!

Apple Dumplings

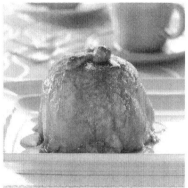

Calories: 367 Fat: 7g Protein: 2g Sugar: 5g
Prep: 15 minutes
Servings: 4

Ingredients:

- 2 tbsp. melted coconut oil
- 2 puff pastry sheets
- 1 tbsp. brown sugar
- 2 tbsp. raisins
- 2 small apples of choice

Directions:

- Ensure your air fryer is preheated to 356 degrees.

- Core and peel apples and mix with raisins and sugar.

- Place a bit of apple mixture into puff pastry sheets and brush sides with melted coconut oil.

- Place into air fryer. Cook 25 minutes, turning halfway through. Will be golden when done.

Air Fryer Chocolate Cake

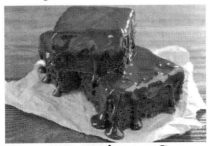

Calories: 378 Fat: 9g Protein: 4g Sugar: 5g
Prep: 5 minutes
Servings: 8-10

Ingredients:
- ½ C. hot water
- 1 tsp. vanilla
- ¼ C. olive oil
- ½ C. almond milk
- 1 egg
- ½ tsp. salt
- ¾ tsp. baking soda
- ¾ tsp. baking powder
- ½ C. unsweetened cocoa powder
- 2 C. almond flour
- 1 C. brown sugar

Directions:
- Preheat your air fryer to 356 degrees.
- Stir all dry ingredients together. Then stir in wet ingredients. Add hot water last.
- The batter will be thin, no worries.
- Pour cake batter into a pan that fits into the fryer. Cover with foil and poke holes into the foil.
- Bake 35 minutes.
- Discard foil and then bake another 10 minutes.

Easy Air Fryer Donuts

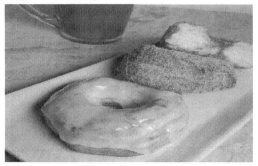

Calories: 209 Fat: 4g Protein: 0g Sugar: 3g
Prep: 5 minutes
Servings: 8

Ingredients:
- Pinch of allspice
- 4 tbsp. dark brown sugar
- ½ - 1 tsp. cinnamon
- 1/3 C. granulated sweetener
- 3 tbsp. melted coconut oil
- 1 can of biscuits

Directions:
- Mix allspice, sugar, sweetener, and cinnamon together.
- Take out biscuits from can and with a circle cookie cutter, cut holes from centers and place into air fryer.
- Cook 5 minutes at 350 degrees. As batches are cooked, use a brush to coat with melted coconut oil and dip each into sugar mixture.
- Serve warm!

Chocolate Soufflé for Two

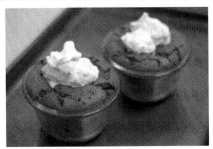

Calories: 238 Fat: 6g Protein: 1g Sugar: 4g
Prep: 15 minutes
Servings: 2

Ingredients:
- 2 tbsp. almond flour
- ½ tsp. vanilla
- 3 tbsp. sweetener
- 2 separated eggs
- ¼ C. melted coconut oil
- 3 ounces of semi-sweet chocolate, chopped

Directions:
- Brush coconut oil and sweetener onto ramekins.
- Melt coconut oil and chocolate together. Beat egg yolks well, adding vanilla and sweetener. Stir in flour and ensure there are no lumps.
- Preheat fryer to 330 degrees.
- Whisk egg whites till they reach peak state and fold them into chocolate mixture.
- Pour batter into ramekins and place into the fryer.
- Cook 14 minutes.
- Serve with powdered sugar dusted on top.

Apple Hand Pies

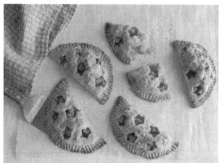

Calories: 278 Fat: 10g Protein: 5g Sugar: 4g
Prep: 5 minutes
Servings: 6

Ingredients:

- 15-ounces no-sugar-added apple pie filling
- 1 store-bought crust

Directions:

- Lay out pie crust and slice into equal-sized squares.
- Place 2 tbsp. filling into each square and seal crust with a fork.
- Place into the fryer. Cook 8 minutes at 390 degrees until golden in color.

Blueberry Lemon Muffins

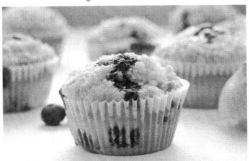

Calories: 317 Fat: 11g Protein: 3g Sugar: 5g
Prep: 10 minutes
Servings: 12

Ingredients:

- 1 tsp. vanilla
- Juice and zest of 1 lemon
- 2 eggs
- 1 C. blueberries
- ½ C. cream
- ¼ C. avocado oil
- ½ C. monk fruit
- 2 ½ C. almond flour

Directions:

- Mix monk fruit and flour together.
- In another bowl, mix vanilla, egg, lemon juice, and cream together. Add mixtures together and blend well.
- Spoon batter into cupcake holders. Place in air fryer. Bake 10 minutes at 320 degrees, checking at 6 minutes to ensure you don't overbake them.

Sweet Cream Cheese Wontons

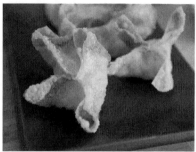

Calories: 303 Fat: 3g Protein: 0.5g Sugar: 4g
Prep: 10 minutes
Makes 16-20

Ingredients:
- 1 egg mixed with a bit of water
- Wonton wrappers
- ½ C. powdered erythritol
- 8 ounces softened cream cheese
- Olive oil

Directions:
- Mix sweetener and cream cheese together.
- Lay out 4 wontons at a time and cover with a dish towel to prevent drying out.
- Place ½ of a teaspoon of cream cheese mixture into each wrapper.
- Dip finger into egg/water mixture and fold diagonally to form a triangle. Seal edges well.
- Repeat with remaining ingredients.
- Place filled wontons into air fryer and cook 5 minutes at 400 degrees, shaking halfway through cooking.

Air Fryer Cinnamon Rolls

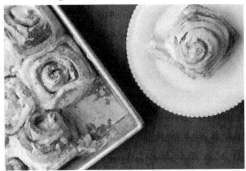

Calories: 390 Fat: 8g Protein: 1g Sugar: 7g
Prep: 15 minutes
Servings: 8

Ingredients:
- 1 ½ tbsp. cinnamon
- ¾ C. brown sugar
- ¼ C. melted coconut oil
- 1 pound frozen bread dough, thawed

Glaze:

- ½ tsp. vanilla
- 1 ¼ C. powdered erythritol
- 2 tbsp. softened ghee
- 4 ounces softened cream cheese

Directions:

- Lay out bread dough and roll out into a rectangle. Brush melted ghee over dough and leave a 1-inch border along edges.

- Mix cinnamon and sweetener together and then sprinkle over dough.

- Roll dough tightly and slice into 8 pieces. Let sit 1-2 hours to rise.
- To make the glaze, simply mix ingredients together till smooth.
- Once rolls rise, place into air fryer and cook 5 minutes at 350 degrees.
- Serve rolls drizzled in cream cheese glaze. Enjoy!

French Toast Bites

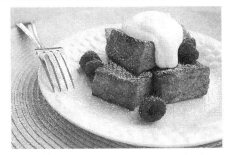

Calories: 289 Fat: 11g Protein: 0g Sugar: 4g
Prep: 5 minutes
Servings: 8

Ingredients:
- Almond milk
- Cinnamon
- Sweetener
- 3 eggs
- 4 pieces wheat bread

Directions:
- Preheat air fryer to 360 degrees.

- Whisk eggs and thin out with almond milk.

- Mix 1/3 cup of sweetener with lots of cinnamon.

- Tear bread in half, ball up pieces and press together to form a ball.

- Soak bread balls in egg and then roll into cinnamon sugar, making sure to thoroughly coat.

- Place coated bread balls into air fryer and bake 15 minutes.

Baked Apple

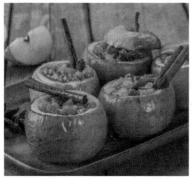

Calories: 199 Fat: 9g Protein: 1g Sugar: 3g
Prep: 10 minutes
Servings: 4

Ingredients:
- ¼ C. water
- ¼ tsp. nutmeg
- ¼ tsp. cinnamon
- 1 ½ tsp. melted ghee
- 2 tbsp. raisins
- 2 tbsp. chopped walnuts
- 1 medium apple

Directions:
- Preheat your air fryer to 350 degrees.
- Slice apple in half and discard some of the flesh from the center.
- Place into frying pan.
- Mix remaining ingredients together except water. Spoon mixture to the middle of apple halves.
- Pour water over filled apples.
- Place pan with apple halves into air fryer, bake 20 minutes.

Cinnamon Sugar Roasted Chickpeas

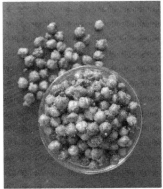

Calories: 111 Fat: 19g Protein: 16g Sugar: 5g
Prep: 10 minutes
Servings: 2

Ingredients:

- 1 tbsp. sweetener
- 1 tbsp. cinnamon
- 1 C. chickpeas

Directions:

- Preheat air fryer to 390 degrees.

- Rinse and drain chickpeas.

- Mix all ingredients together and add to air fryer.

- Cook 10 minutes.

Cinnamon Fried Bananas

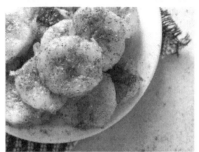

Calories: 219 Fat: 10g Protein: 3g Sugar: 5g
Prep: 5 minutes
Servings: 2-3

Ingredients:

- 1 C. panko breadcrumbs
- 3 tbsp. cinnamon
- ½ C. almond flour
- 3 egg whites
- 8 ripe bananas
- 3 tbsp. vegan coconut oil

Directions:

- Heat coconut oil and add breadcrumbs. Mix around 2-3 minutes until golden. Pour into bowl.
- Peel and cut bananas in half. Roll each bananas half into flour, eggs, and crumb mixture. Place into air fryer.
- Cook 10 minutes at 280 degrees.
- A great addition to a healthy banana split!

Conclusion

I want to congratulate you for making it to the last page of *Healthy Air Fryer Recipes*!

I hope that you found this one-of-a-kind cookbook to be valuable in regard to creating a better version of yourself! There are many ways that you can make the best better in your physical life that spills into other aspects as well.

I hope that this book assisted you in gaining the confidence to purchase an air fryer and uses it on a regular basis! If you wish to become more fit, you must be willing to give up fast food and junk food, for that is no way to fuel the one body you get in this life. I hope that the chapters you have newly absorbed help you to achieve your goals, whatever they may be.

The next step is to put the information you have learned to the test in your life! Pick out a few recipes that caught your eye and make it a priority to take that first step to a better life by making and enjoying them!

If you found this book to be beneficial and valuable, please take a moment from creating delicious meals with your air fryer to head over to Amazon and leave a review! It is always appreciated!

20855634R00084

Made in the USA
San Bernardino, CA
29 December 2018